Kundalini

A Beginner's Guide to Kundalini Awakening

Lauren Lingard

Table of Contents

Introduction 1

Chapter One: What Is Kundalini? 4

Chapter Two: The Mystical History of this Ancient Practice 11

Chapter Three: How to 'awaken' Kundalini and what will that feel like? 16

Chapter Four: A Kundalini Yoga Practice for Beginners 21

Chapter Five: Understanding the subtle energies we activate with Kundalini Breathwork 35

Chapter Six: Kundalini You 44

Conclusion 55

Introduction

Finding Your 'Serpent' Power

Yoga has become so popular in the Western world you can probably step into your local gym and book a drop-in class. You can find an abundance of yoga courses on YouTube and just as many glam-looking yoga teachers on Instagram who offer holiday retreats centered on an enjoyable daily yoga practice. But what very few people - many teachers and practitioners alike - truly understand is that the type of yoga most people are practicing is simply a 'warm up' for another type altogether: Kundalini yoga.

Kundalini is just shorthand for the full Sanskrit name of this mystical practice, which is **Kundalini Shakti**, and in that name lies a clue as to what this practice is all about. Kundain, in Sanskrit, means circular and, is often used as a noun for a snake and so loosely translated, Kundalini means snake. Shakti is the Hindu name for a divine form of female energy and so if you put the two together, you can figure out what Kundalini Yoga must be about.

All yoga practices - including the special breathing techniques (*pranayama*) you will learn and even the chants and hand gestures (*mudras*) has a specific purpose and even if nobody has ever told you this, that purpose is to first align and rebalance the unseen flow of energy (life force) through your body before starting the all-important task of awakening the dormant energy known as Kundalini or, if you prefer, 'the serpent power.'

I will explain, as you work your way through the book, more about why this will be beneficial to your physical, psychological, and spiritual wellbeing and, just as importantly, show you how to awaken your Kundalini; a process that will change your life.

We've just seen how Kundalini relates to the divine feminine energy called Shakti, but this does not mean Kundalini yoga is only for women - this energy is available to and a part of us all, so whatever gender you identify with, don't worry. You have the same potential as the person on the yoga mat alongside you.

With all yoga practices, a student can take their understanding and then the practice itself as deeply as they wish and feel comfortable doing, but of all the different schools of yoga, Kundalini yoga makes no secret of its goal - the awakening of Kundalini energy - and so it is described as the most spiritual of all the different types of yoga. If deepening your spiritual beliefs and understanding are your goal, rather than simply improving fitness and trimming your waistline, then Kundalini yoga will be an excellent choice for you.

Where other more dynamic yoga practices such as ashtanga or 'hot' yoga place more emphasis on fitness and burning calories, Kundalini is more overtly esoteric. People who choose Kundalini yoga for its unashamed emphasis on being primarily a spiritual practice, (although, since it is yoga, it is also one that will boost your overall health and wellbeing too), often signal this choice by wearing white for their yoga classes.

You will learn yoga postures (*asanas*) that encourage the awakening of Kundalini, but you will also learn chanting and meditation and *mudras (*hand gestures) and even clever ways of locking energy into various parts of the body (bandhas) to achieve the goal of raising the Kundalini energy, but you will also quickly understand this is a slow process and not something you can rush or put a deadline on achieving. This means you will also learn the important lesson that in life, the journey is just as important as the goal!

In this book, I will take you on that journey so that by the time you read the last word of the last chapter, you will feel confident this is the right type of yoga for you and you will know what you are looking for and be able to assess how you are progressing in either your private practice or a yoga class, whichever way you choose of deepening your practice and awakening your serpent power.

Chapter One: What Is Kundalini?

"The primary aim of Kundalini is to awaken the full potential of human awareness in each individual; that is, recognize our awareness, refine that awareness, and expand that awareness to our unlimited Self. Clear any inner duality, create the power to deeply listen, cultivate inner stillness, and prosper and deliver excellence in all that we do."

-Kundalini Research Institute

We know from the meaning of the words, Kundalini Shakti, that Kundalini is a special energy that we can use yoga - both postures and breathwork - to awaken. We know too that until we choose to commit to this as a goal, the Kundalini will remain dormant in the body, which means all the potential powers and benefits it can bring us will remain dormant too.

So, the first thing to understand as we step onto the Kundalini path is that it is a path, a spiritual one, and that it calls for a commitment from us.

You won't achieve your goal of awakening your Kundalini by dipping in and out of the practices I will share with you in this book but, as with most things, little and often is going to be the most beneficial approach to getting the most out of your Kundalini practice, especially when you are just starting and stepping on to your yoga mat as a beginner. In fact, as a beginner, we need to park all thoughts of Kundalini to one side for a while and make sure we understand how, in yoga, the Kundalini energy works with the *prana* (life force) that is not dormant but flows through us keeping us alive.

Prana is not the same as the breath, although in yoga, especially Kundalini yoga, we learn how to use special breathing techniques to balance and even direct the flow of *prana*. If you want to understand the important difference between the two, then think about this: You can hold your breath, and remain alive for several minutes but in yoga, we believe if your *prana* stopped flowing for even a single second your life would end. That's why we also call it the life force.

The energy (prana) that is the divine female energy of Kundalini lies dormant until we do the work to awaken it, so there must be another energy (*pranic*) field that is already awake and keeping us alive. There is, and this energy field flows through and between special energy centers known as chakras.

If you are already familiar with the chakra energy system from studying other esoteric traditions or healing practices, it is still worth looking here at our yogic understanding of these centers; what they are called, what they are doing, and why they are important in helping us to awaken our serpent power.

In yoga, we describe the chakras as spinning 'wheels of light' and imagine these energy centers are firing our 'sparks of light' (*prana*) to flow through and around the body. It is important to remember this is an esoteric idea and so these are not physical centers (like organs or cells) that can be seen by the naked eye or under the microscope. Like thoughts and feelings and mood, they play a significant role in our holistic wellbeing but work mystically, which means we must adopt a similar mystical approach to working with them.

That's why we use breath, meditation, intuition, and a practice - yoga - that has been used for millennia to show us how to achieve a union of body, mind, and soul with Divine Consciousness.

Let's look now at the seven major chakras we will work with later in the book to signal the Kundalini energy that the time is right, and we are ready for it to rise in us and help us reach our full potential.

The Seven Major Chakras

In chakra work, we always start at the bottom of the body at what is called the 'root' chakra and work our way up to the 'crown chakra at the top of the head. You can imagine this as a straight line that follows the alignment of your spine and which allows energy (*prana*) to run up and down it between the chakra centers which can then fire that energy off to where it is needed and, once you become proficient at this inner work, where you deliberately send it.

Another way to imagine your chakra centers and how they connect is to see, in your mind's eye, a long, strong thread that strings together seven beautiful and precious gemstones, each stone representing a specific energy center (chakra).

So, let's look now at each center and learn where it sits in the body and what it does.

The Root Chakra - Muladhara

The clue is in the name and so the 'root' chakra is at the base (root) of your spinal column. This is the energy center that represents your safety, security, and resilience. The energy here is the energy that will ground you, especially when external life challenges are coming your way, which means you need to stand steadfast.

Where is it?

If you were born a female, the root chakra is behind your cervix at the bottom of your spinal column. If you are biologically male, you need to imagine this energy center as being located midway between your scrotum and your anus.

The Sacral Chakra - Svadhisthana

Move your finger to your naval and then drop it to just below, and you will be in the place of the sacral chakra which governs how you interact with the world and in particular, your creative energies, including your sexual (reproductive) energy. This center, when balanced, helps you regulate your own emotions and 'pick up' on the feelings of others so you can respond appropriately.

Where is it?

Use your finger to feel for the base of your spinal column and find the place known as your coccyx or tailbone. This is the home of the sacral chakra.

The Solar Plexus Chakra - Manipura

Unlike with the sacral chakra, you can't really 'feel' this one out with your fingers because it lies in your stomach, where it oversees your self-esteem and your self-confidence. When this energy center tips out of balance, you may feel you are losing control in life and over what is happening to you.

Where is it?

You can imagine this chakra as one of the linked gemstones we talked about before, so in your mind's eye, imagine a bright light that sits in the core of your being, just above your navel.

The Heart Chakra - Anhata

This is the energy center that allows you to be the loving person you were born to be and someone who can accept love from others. Unfortunately, this means this is also the energy center that can become seriously unbalanced when hearts are broken, feelings are hurt, and trust is broken.

Where is it?
Put the middle fingers of your right hand on the breastbone in the middle of your chest and, if you are a biological female, between the breasts. Your heart chakra lies not over your heart, as you may have expected, but right in the middle of your chest.

The Throat Chakra - Vishuddu

If speaking out and allowing yourself to communicate authentically is difficult for you, then maybe this energy center is blocked and out of balance. If you have ever had a frightening dream where (in the dream) you try to call out but there is no sound, this is what a blocked throat chakra would feel like. Or worse, you make sounds, but they make no sense!

Where is it?
Put the index finger of your right hand on the middle of your throat and gently feel for the 'lump' that is your voice box. This is where the throat chakra lies. When you are emotionally upset or distressed, you can feel this area tightening as you struggle to manage your emotions.

The Third Eye Chakra - Ajna

You may already have heard talk of the mystical 'Third Eye' and wondered what that was all about? It is simply another name for the 6th of the seven major chakras and is the center that governs your gut instincts, your imagination, and even your psychic powers!

Where is it?
This energy center sits right at the top of the spinal column. We can't feel that, but we can put the index finger of the right hand in the middle of the forehead, at the level of the eyebrows, and this is where the Third Eye sits.

The Crown Chakra - Sahasrara

This is the chakra you can think of as your 'crowning glory.' This is the important energy center that links you with your Higher Self, your life purpose, and all the spiritual aspects of your being, and so this then is the eventual destination of the Kundalini energy you will learn to awaken and raise in this book.

Where is it?

Imagine the last of the seven chakra 'gemstones' we are talking about here, sitting right in the center and on top of your head. You can visualize this chakra as blazing with white light and shining the brightest of them all.

Kundalini - Raising the Serpent Power

It has been important to work our way through the seven major chakra energy centers and to visualize, in our mind's eye, where they are located because Kundalini yoga works to achieve two specific goals:

Goal (1): Awaken Kundalini Shakti

Goal (2) Raise Kundalini Shakti

We have learned that until we decide to achieve these goals and learn how we can both awaken and raise Kundalini energy, it will remain dormant, and we will miss out on reaching our full spiritual, psychological, physical, and emotional wellbeing potential. Understanding the chakra pathway is crucial to understanding (and visualizing) how it is we will raise the awakened Kundalini energy. By now, as you will have guessed, we will use these same linked energy pathways to lift and raise Kundalini energy through the body to the spiritual energy center in the crown chakra.

Chapter Summary

- We have discovered Kundalini Shakti (to give it its full name) is the energy of the Divine Female which lies dormant in us all, male and female, until we decide to awaken it.

- Once we have awakened this energy - also known as our Serpent Power - we can use it as a force for the greater good, in our own lives and the lives of others, but only if we learn how to raise it through the body

- In this chapter, we have seen how we will use the chakra pathways - and the chakra energy centers themselves - to help raise Kundalini

In the next chapter, we will look at the once-hidden history and the true meaning of Kundalini energy and learn more about what happens when it awakens.

Chapter Two: The Mystical History of this Ancient Practice

"It is everyone's birthright to be healthy, happy, and holy, and the practice of Kundalini Yoga is the way to claim that birthright."

While the exact origins of Kundalini Yoga have been lost in the mists of time, the first written references to this practice of raising the divine energy force appeared in the sacred Vedic texts known as the Upanishads at around 1000 B.C.

The word '*Upanishads*' translates to: "*Sitting down to hear the spiritual teachings of the Master.*"

In the Eastern esoteric traditions like yoga, students learned at the feet of the Gurus or Masters, and understood they were receiving wisdom that had been passed, orally at first, down the ages from guru to disciple and master to student for eons. A big part of that understanding and tradition was (is) that the student accepts the master's wisdom, word for word. There is no arguing and debating back and forth (which would likely be the case today in the Western world) but a deep reverence for the honor of being allowed to hear these spiritual teachings.

Today, with Kundalini, that has not changed. There is still a sense of it being an honor and a privilege to learn from those that have gone before and are further along the yogic path of understanding than you are, and people often remark that the inherent reverence of a Kundalini yoga class or private practice feels more like a religious temple ritual than a fitness class.

This reverence has deep roots because, for thousands of years, Kundalini yoga was deliberately kept secret and only passed from the guru to those disciples deemed worthy after many years of training and initiations. And it remained that way, a closely guarded secret of those considered the spiritual elite, until 1968 when Yogi Bahjan arrived in Toronto, Canada, and saw, during a weekend meditation class in Los Angeles, that it was his duty to teach Kundalini yoga to the West.

It has been reported that he saw in the hippie counterculture of that time a yearning from young people to make a more meaningful spiritual connection with the Divine but that it appeared the only way they could achieve that was by using drugs.

Yogi Bhajan knew he could offer a different and healthier route to the same destination and so he put down roots in Los Angeles and started his first Kundalini yoga class with the proclamation that everyone may be" healthy, happy and holy" and that the practice of Kundalini (not illegal drugs) was the way to claim that birthright. Yogi Bhajan set up the 3HO (Healthy, Happy, Holy Organization) and the Kundalini Research Institute. He wrote books and was the founder of International Peace Prayer Day. He believed passionately that we all have a responsibility to help improve society through mindfulness and compassion, and he saw Kundalini yoga as a way of teaching and making practical spirituality a reality for everyone.

Yogi Bhajan shared with his followers five key mantras, the meaning of which, although the language he uses (e.g., cosmos) is very much of its time, are still relevant to our practice today. They are:

Yogi Bhajan's Five Mantras
- Recognize that the other person is you
- There is a way through every block
- When the time is on you, start, and the pressure will be off
- Understand through compassion or you will misunderstand the times
- Vibrate the cosmos and the cosmos shall clear the path.

Kundalini is the Yoga of Awareness

Kundalini yoga is often described as the 'yoga of awareness' and so you might ask awareness of what? The simple response is that it is a new awareness that you will gain regarding the following core yogic beliefs:

1. God is not 'some bearded bloke' hovering above you in the sky that is just too busy and disconnected from you to bother with your complaints and issues

2. You are not the Ego Personality you have developed to present to the world — the real you, is a being without ego, which we refer to as The Higher Self

3. The purpose of Kundalini yoga is to recognize the divine inside of you and unleash it to allow you to reveal your Higher Self, and through that Self, help, inspire, and heal others and thus fulfill your life's purpose

Why have I heard Kundalini can be dangerous?

"Because many people are confused by Kundalini's real nature, we must do more to define it accurately, starting with what it is not. For example, it isn't devil worship or a supernatural cult. Neither is it a religion nor a sect. It's a biological process. You can't be converted to Kundalini any more than you can be converted to a heart attack or an orgasm; they just happen. That's the nature of biological processes: They just happen."

— JJ Semple, The Biology of Consciousness: Case Studies in Kundalini

Whenever something comes out of the 'shadows' there is always the risk it will be misunderstood and that because of those misunderstandings, people will find it threatening. At first, when Yogi Bhajan began sharing the spiritual teachings and practices of Kundalini Yoga with Westerners, it would also have angered those gurus who firmly believed it was not a practice to be shared with the 'unprepared' masses, and so a disinformation campaign would have been unleashed. Better to scare people away than risk modification or even a perceived abuse of such a protected esoteric practice. Although they seem unrelated, you can think of this as being like the way some countries that export wine to the rest of the world keep the 'good stuff' back for themselves because the principle is the same. It is not right or wrong, it just is.

But there is another reason that you may have heard Kundalini Yoga is to be avoided which has nothing to do with misunderstandings or misinformation, and that is because the practice can trigger some unexpected 'experiences' for some people. Until you step onto the path you don't know if that could be you.

Unexpected 'experiences' sounds scary but just means you may have feelings and emotional outbursts that will shock you, and this is because as you awaken the Kundalini energy, you will trigger raw emotions and some of these may come from negative experiences you have had. Some practitioners have experienced a reaction they describe as similar to panic and some even tell of outbursts that to others look like drug-induced behaviors or even psychosis, but these reactions are rare and are usually the result of someone who has not laid the foundations or prepared the groundwork for the awakening of Kundalini in a safe, slow, and proper way.

I said, in the introduction, this is not a practice to be rushed, and sometimes the negativity that can surround Kundalini yoga comes from the frustration that even after months and years of practice the student feels nothing has changed and nothing seems to happen. It is then probably easier to blame the teachings themselves than the fact there may still be 'blockages' the student needs to work on to awaken the Kundalini.

Happily, most people who find their way to these beautiful teachings and this deeply spiritual practice report feeling happier, more balanced, more creative, and more compassionate towards others than they have felt for years!

Chapter Summary

- Kundalini Yoga was unknown in the Western world until the late 1960s; and only shared with the elite in India until that time.

- This once secretive practice is known as the 'yoga of awareness' with the key awareness being that the divine energy inside of you (Kundalini Shakti) is the same as the Divine energy that made you.

- Kundalini yoga can help you shed your limiting Ego Personality and connect to your Higher Self

In the next chapter, we will explore some ways in which Kundalini can awaken and what that can feel like when it happens.

Chapter Three: How to 'awaken' Kundalini and what will that feel like?

"There are two energies inside you: Architect (he) and Mystic (she). He needs to plan; he needs how and why of everything. She just watches things unfold; the universe shows her its most mysterious and magical depths. She can accept him because human planning is just a small part of universal magic. But he feels threatened by her. So, she is asleep inside you."

-Shunya

What must happen for Kundalini energy to awaken?

While your Kundalini yoga practice will focus on postures (*asanas*) to align and balance the chakras, breathing techniques to direct *prana* (energy), and meditation, you can expect a range of different activities as part of a Kundalini *kryia* — including dancing, chanting, stretching, yelling, and even running.

A *kryia* is the name we give to all the practices we include in a Kundalini session or class. These will include *asana* (posture), *pranayama* (breathwork), *mantra* (chanting), *bandhas* (energy locks), and *mudra* (hand gestures). Each of these elements is used to create movement and change in the body and the mind, and there are so many Kundalini *kryias* (literally, thousands of them) you can find a *kryia* to help you become less fearful, or to strengthen your ankles, or to refine your sexuality.

This is also the point where you need to understand that whilst you and I may work our way through the same *kryia* on our yoga mats in class, our individual experience of that *kryia* will be unique to us: you won't feel the same way either during or afterward that I do.

Remember, the goal of the Kundalini *kryia* is not to perform a perfect *asana* (posture) or outperform everyone else in the class; the goal is to use these movements and patterns to change your energy, open the chakra energy centers, and raise the Kundalini energy through the chakras to the crown of the head. Remember too, you cannot rush this, and whilst some practitioners report a spontaneous awakening and arising of the Kundalini energy, these people are the exception to the rule. For most of us, it takes months, even years of dedicated practice, which is a good thing because as we can see, a sudden unleashing of the Kundalini energy could be an overwhelming experience. It's far better for the energy to awaken when you are ready physically, mentally, and spiritually.

How will it feel when this happens?

We have now seen that the underlying purpose behind Kundalini yoga and practicing Kundalini *kryias* is to awaken the Kundalini Shakti (divine feminie) energy and allow it to rise through the open chakras so we can discover our true identities.

Until we do this, it can feel as if we are sleepwalking through our lives and failing to find our true purpose.

As Kundalini awakens, you may feel sensations and experience symptoms that you have not had before. When Kundalini arises, it itself won't cause these kinds of problems. What causes these issues is when the Kundalini is trying to rise and move up through the chakras and it becomes blocked. What you will then experience is actually the result of those chakra blockages, rather than the impact of this new energy itself.

The whole point of awakening your Kundalini is to allow you to connect with your Higher Self and to reveal your true identity to yourself, so it is important to pay attention to these blockages and to do the work - using your yoga practice and techniques - to keep your chakras open and balanced and ensure they stay open and balanced.

Once the path is clear for Kundalini Shakti to rise, here are some signs that will signal she is on the move and some changes you may now experience:

- If the awakening of the previously dormant Kundalini is very sudden for you, then you may experience strong physical signs including tremors, shakes, seeing flashing colors, panic attacks, and even the feeling of a sudden rush of energy. This is rare though because for most people the awakening is a slow process.

- You may go through an intense period of low mood at the start of these changes and experience anxiety, depression, and despair for a while. Sit through it, it will pass.

- You want to try new things.

- You find the courage to change what's not working for you anymore; you may leave relationships and jobs and set your sights on pastures new.

- You may notice more coincidences and synchronicities in your life. You may even feel you are blessed by miracles happening in your life.

- You enjoy more support from others, especially from unexpected places.

- More compassion towards others.

- Greater sensitivity to external stimuli, including food, other people and their energy and media bombardment, especially violence in films or news reporting.

- Simple sense of your life purpose and your dignity.

The important thing, whatever you experience, is to stay in your body, not your head. Your nervous system is expanding to accommodate this new influx of energy (Kundalini Shakti) and will become more sensitive. Don't see this as a problem or a weakness, it is a necessity to allow the full potential of this energy to express itself.

The feelings you have are likely to be intensified at the start of the day, when you awake, and just before you go to sleep at night. Again, stay in your body. Don't allow your mind to run away obsessing about what is happening or to introduce fear into the mix. Decrease the stressful elements of your everyday life to give your body the time and space it needs to change the availability of the Kundalini energy.

Focus now on a daily Kundalini yoga practice and meditation and try to connect with like-minded people either in your local community or failing that, online. Remember, you are changing, and change always comes with discomfort. You will feel as if you are 'shedding a skin' to become a new person. It is not a new person stepping into the place once occupied by you, it is the Higher Self we talked about as being the version of you that you will meet once the Kundalini has been awakened and its passages up through the open chakras is facilitated.

Do not feel you are alone. Worldly events now move at such a pace there has been, especially recently, a collective awakening. You are not alone. As your Kundalini awakens and rises, take comfort in knowing you are among these awakened souls who will no longer accept injustice, greed, and war for its own sake.

Chapter Summary

- Kundalini yoga *kryias* are set practices that encourage the awakening of Kundalini in a safe and prepared way

- We have learned that for the Kundalini energy to rise, the chakra centers need to be open and balanced to facilitate its path

- Once this starts, you will not experience life in the same way, want the same things, or be the same person because you will become more aligned with your Higher Self

In the next chapter, we will learn a Kundalini *kryia* designed to start this process.

Chapter Four: A Kundalini Yoga Practice for Beginners

We have seen how a single Kundalini practice session or class will comprise multiple elements that all have their roots in the spiritual and philosophical ancient traditions of yoga - including *asana* (posture), *pranayama* (breathwork), meditation, chanting, *bandha* (energy locks), and *mudra* (sacred hand gestures). Together, these make up the Kundalini *kryia* that we can practice at home, or in class.

So, in this practical introduction to Kundalini yoga, we will work through one practice from each element that is suited to a beginner's practice. Remember though, before you start, that Kundalini yoga is the yoga of awareness and that your experience of a kryia will not be the same as someone else's. The most important thing in any yoga practice — and particularly a Kundalini practice — is to listen to your body and to do what works for you.

If this means adapting this suggested practice, that is fine. However, if you need a shorter practice session, then shorten the time you spend with each element, and don't be tempted to cut corners by ditching one or two elements entirely. To do that would wreck the pre-planned and carefully designed 'flow' of the *kryia* which has begun to awaken the Kundalini energy and which, as you master it, will make sense to you not only on a physical level but on a spiritual one too.

A Kundalini Practice for Beginners

You can think of this Beginner's Kundalini Kryia as a 4-Step practice which will take about 30 minutes. But don't rush through it. If you want to take longer on your mat and take more time to work through this Kryia, do so. We are not on the clock!

Step (1) Welcome Mantra chant

A mantra is simply a sacred sound or word that we repeat in a yoga practice to reduce negative energy and lift the mood. You can use a mantra practice on its own to banish headaches and depression, but for this session, we are using a mantra or chant to tune in to our Higher Selves and to open the session.

Every Kundalini yoga class opens with the same sacred mantra which is:

"Om Namo Guru Dev Namo"

Translated from these Sanskrit words, this mantra means:

'*I bow to the Creative Wisdom. I bow to the Divine Wisdom within.*'

We repeat this powerful and sacred statement to connect us at the start of our practice to what is called the 'Golden Chani' which simply means the teachings of yoga and the teachers and students who have gone before us or who are ahead of us on the path. You can also think of it as connecting you to the wise tradition and mystical legacy of yoga through the eons. Take a minute to find some examples of someone chanting this mantra online so you can see how they settle into this mantra.

When you are ready to start, sit cross-legged (or if you are flexible enough, in the lotus position) on your yoga mat and close your eyes. Settle yourself by breathing in deeply through the nose, hold the breath for a count of four and then slowly breathe out, again through the nose and not the mouth. Do this three or four times to help you bring your awareness inside and to settle and calm your body to prepare for your Kundalini yoga practice.

When you feel calm and settled, rub your hands together to wake the nerve endings in them and to balance the left and right hemispheres of the brain, and then place your hands in the prayer position (mudra). Now bring them together and press your thumbs into the center of your chest.

Close your eyes, inhale through your nose, and repeat the welcome chant, three times.

Beginner's tip: *You may feel shy about chanting out loud at first, so practice silently in your mind until you are comfortable with the sounds you will make and feel ready to unleash your chanting voice.*

Step (2) Asanas to open Muladhara (root) chakra

We know that the Kundalini energy lies dormant - like a coiled snake - at the base of the spine where we also find the root or Muladhara chakra, so these are asanas (postures) that awaken the energy in this region, open that chakra ready for the ascent of Kundalini, and prepare the whole body for the energy to awaken.

(i) Sufi grind

Stay sitting cross-legged in a comfortable position on your yoga mat. Prop your hips up with a yoga block or a cushion to raise them above your knees and prevent the back from feeling strain. As you breathe in, lean your upper torso forwards, and then circle from your waist to the right and use the center of your body to make a circle back to the front again. You lean forward on the inhale to start the circle and exhale as you allow the body to lean back. Remember to always breathe through the nose.

Hold your shins with your hands as you circle, and feel the shoulders loosen and relax as your body settles into this circular motion. Once you are comfortable making this circular motion, you can add a mantra and chant (or say silently to yourself) '**Sat**' as you lean forward on the inhale and '**Nam**' as you roll from your waist backward to complete the full circle. This mantra loosely translates to you saying that you are centered in your truth. Remember, too, you can use a mantra to train a wandering mind and regain focus throughout your practice.

Make five circles in a clockwise direction and then reverse to make five circles in an anti-clockwise direction.

Once you stop, bring your torso back to the center position, keep your eyes closed and take several more, deep breaths. Notice how this posture has changed your energy and your mood.

Beginner's tip: *Do not strain to make a circular motion if your back feels very stiff. Instead, practice rocking slowly forwards and backward by bending from the middle of the torso and try to synchronize your body's movements with the breath; forwards on the inhale, and backward as you breathe out again. This will help loosen the back so eventually, you will be able to 'circle' from the waist causing no strain.*

(ii) Spine Flex

Stay seated but remove the yoga block or cushion if it feels more comfortable to do this asana without having the hips at a higher level than the knees. Close your eyes. Keep your chin up and aligned with the floor but as you inhale, push your chest forward and allow your spine to curve inwards. As you exhale, bring the chest and torso back and allow the bottom of the spine to flex outwards.

Settle into a rhythmic rocking motion and as you rock forwards chant '**Sat**' and as you rock backward chant "**Nam.**'

Once you get the hang of the rocking motion that flexes the spine, you can exhale more forcibly, but again do this through the nose.

You will feel your entire body warming up as you repeat the rocking and this special yogic breathing technique. Rock as fast or as slowly as you like. Keep your shoulders and jaw relaxed.

Rock for at least a minute, or longer if you like. Once you stop, bring your torso back to the center position, keep your eyes closed and take several more, deep breaths. Notice how this posture has changed your energy and your mood.

(iii) Skandh Chakra (shoulder rotation)

Stay seated on your mat and bring your hands to your shoulders, placing your thumbs behind your shoulders and your fingers in front. Close your eyes, engage your core abdominal muscles and bring your awareness to the shoulder socket joints. You are going to use the elbows to make big circles that rotate both shoulder joints. Inhales as you lift the elbows towards your ears and exhale as you rotate them back and down again. Repeat this five times and then reverse the circle, still using your elbows to make the rotation. As you reverse, notice how it feels once the shoulder joints loosen and open up. Notice too now the back muscles love this movement, especially if you have spent all day hunched over a computer keyboard or if you have been driving all day.

This exercise opens the chest and works on the heart chakra to keep the loving energy flowing and free.

(iv) Dynamic waist twist

Keep your hands on your shoulders and this time, as you inhale, twist from your waist to the left and as you exhale, come back and pass through the center and twist round back to the right. And as you exhale, you can forcibly push the breath out through your nostrils.

You will find your body naturally settling into the power of this twisting movement which releases tension from your back. Keep your abdominal muscles engaged and as you adopt the synchronized yogic breathing practice (*pranayama*) you will feel your body warming up.

Once you have twisted five times, exhaling to the right, reverse and twist five times more, but exhaling to the left.

Keep your eyes closed throughout and place your awareness near the Third Eye so that as you twist the physical body, you also activate your intuition.

Once you stop, bring your torso back to the center position, keep your eyes closed and take several more, deep breaths. Notice how this posture has changed your energy and your mood.

(v) Supta Udarakarshanasana (sleeping abdominal stretch pose)

Lie on your yoga mat with your feet together and your arms to the sides. Bend the knees and keep the soles of the feet flat on the mat, just in front of the buttocks. Bring your hands up to your head, interlock the fingers and place your hands under your head. Feel your head is supported and cushioned in this hold. Allow the elbows to drop to the mat and as you breathe out, gently lower your legs to the right, keeping your knees and ankles together. As you lower the knees, gently turn the head in the opposite direction, to the left. Feel the deep twist in your spinal column and the deep stretch to the abdominal muscles. Close your eyes and imagine the Kundalini energy lying asleep at the base of the spine and the gentle opening of the Muladhara chakra energy center which will mark the beginning of the Kundalini energy's ascent up through the energy body.

This posture is an excellent counter to sitting and can also help relieve backache and digestive disorders. Once you have relaxed the body into the spinal twist to the right, reverse and do the same to the left, remembering again to turn your head, this time to the right.

You can also make this a more dynamic posture by adopting the same bent knees and hands behind the head. Do this by allowing the body to rock between the two sides, left and right, keeping the elbows on the floor.

(vi) Marjari-asana (cat stretch pose)

Kneel on your mat with your buttocks resting on your heels. Raise your body to bring yourself to a position where you are kneeling on all fours (like a cat) and lean forward, placing your weight onto your hands with your palms flat on your yoga mat. Make sure your hands are in alignment with your knees, and that your arms and thighs are perpendicular to the floor.

As you inhale, raise your head to stretch the throat and as you do so, allow the spine to curve into a concave shape. Allow the abdomen to fully expand and fill your lungs with air. Hold the breath for a count of three and then, as you exhale through the nose, allow your head to drop and the next and throat to relax and stretch your spine in an upward curve. Pull in the stomach muscles and pull in the buttocks too. Hold the breath again for a count of three.

This counts as one round, one inhalation, and one exhalation. Aim to practice five rounds and build up to 10. Try to slow the breath down so the body can settle into this backstretch and counter stretch.

Once you stop, come back to a comfortable sitting position, close your eyes, and take several more, deep breaths. Notice how this practice has changed your energy and your mood.

Beginner's tip: *Do not bend the arms at the elbows but keep them vertical throughout. You can safely practice this posture up to the sixth month of pregnancy.*

(vii) Balasana (pose of the child or baby)

This wonderful and soothing pose serves as a counter to the more vigorous spine bending of the cat pose.

Kneel on your mat and fold your body forward so that your forehead touches the mat itself. Put your arms along the sides of your body and allow them to relax. Bring your awareness to your breath and as you gently exhale, feel your body fold in smaller and all your muscles relax into this posture. If your shoulders have been feeling tense and tight, you can stretch your arms out in front of you, keeping the top of the arm touching the ear on each side. Rest your buttocks on your heels. Close your eyes and let your breath settle you into this soothing posture. If your mind wanders, bring your focus back with the **Sat Nam** mantra. Everything about this *asana* needs to be (and feel) quiet and peaceful.

Once you stop, come back to a comfortable sitting position. Keep your eyes closed and take several more, deep breaths. Notice how this practice has changed your energy and your mood. Tune into the extra energy you have now created with your asana practice and with the opening up of the Muladhara root chakra.

Step (3) Pranayama & Muladhara Bandha
You may have noticed we already used some specific yoga breathwork in the asana practice - remember the torso twist where you swing the shoulders from side to side and exhale more forcibly than you inhale? In this next practice, we take the notion of breath control up a level with a practice known as 'The Fire Breath' or, to give it its proper yogic name, Kapalbhati. You will feel the internal heat being generated almost as soon as you master this technique, which you can also use to energize the mind ready for a busy day at work and to prepare for meditation.

(i) Kapalbhati Pranayama (front brain cleansing)
Yoga teachers describe this (breathwork) practice as 'The Ego Slayer' because you must park all feelings of embarrassment about how you look or sound to others, and even to yourself. It is also known as the 'Breath of Fire.'

Make sure you are sitting comfortably on your yoga mat and use a yoga roll or cushion to raise your hips above the knees so that you can settle into this position for a while and focus on your breathing. Bring your arms up to the side and hold them in a position of 45 degrees.

Inhale deeply through both nostrils, allowing your abdominal muscles to expand, and your lungs to fill with air. Now, exhale sharply and loudly by tensing the abdominal muscles to raise the diaphragm and force the air out of your lungs. Inhaling should be as effortless in this practice as exhaling is strenuous. As you try it, imagine snapping your navel back towards your spine which will ensure you are breathing from your abdomen and not your chest.

Keep count each time you exhale and bring your awareness to your Third Eye as you build up to 10, then 20 then 50 rounds. (A round = one passive inhalation and one exaggerated and forceful exhalation.) Your Breath of Fire can be fast or slow; you can choose what feels right for you. The important thing is consistency.

As you master the mechanics of this breathing technique, you can focus more on the spiritual aspects by keeping your attention on the Third Eye chakra in the middle of your forehead, between your brows. The aim of this pranic practice is, as the common name suggests, to 'cleanse' and calm the mind so you end your practice with an intense feeling of an all-pervading emptiness and calm.

(ii) Moola Bandha

A Bandha is a yogic energy lock and in chapter eight, I will explain more about these, how they change energy flow, and why we use them in a Kundalini practice. For this practice chapter however, which has focused on awakening the energy in the root chakra (Muladhara) I will just focus on the energy lock you can apply in that region of the subtle energy body to ensure the Kundalini energy flows upwards.

To practice Moola Bandha, sit in a comfortable position on your mat and prop your hips above the knees using a yoga block or cushion if that is more comfortable for you.

Close your eyes and bring your awareness to the base of your spine and the Muladhara chakra (also sometimes called Moolahara, hence the name Moola Bandha).

Locate, in your mind's eye, the part of your body known as the perineum which, for women, is between the vagina and the anus, and for males, between the scrotum and the anus.

If you have ever practiced pelvic floor exercises, then you have already done something very similar to applying an energy lock in the root chakra. The difference here is we learn to hold the lock whilst keeping the rest of the body relaxed. And then, once we have mastered that, we can apply the lock, at will, throughout any part of our Kundalini yoga practice.

Stage 1:

- Close the eyes and relax the entire body

- Bring your awareness to your breath and let it rise and fall naturally

- Locate your perineum

- Contract the muscles in that region and feel the pelvic floor rise

- Relax the muscles in that region and feel the pelvic floor drop again

Stage 2:

- Repeat the above contraction of the pelvic floor muscles but do it more deliberately and slowly and try to keep your breathing relaxed and normal.

- Now, hold the contraction for a count of five, before slowly releasing.

- At first, the sphincter muscle that controls the anus will contract too, but as you master Moola Bandha this will stop.

- Do not rush this practice. It can raise the energies quickly unless you are slow and deliberate about mastering it.

- Practice 10 rounds (one round = one contraction and one relaxation) and then stop.

Come back to a comfortable sitting position. Keep your eyes closed and take several more, deep breaths. Notice how this practice has changed your energy and your mood. Tune into the fresh energy you have now created with your asana practice and with the opening up of the Muladhara root chakra.

Step (4) Meditation & Mudra

You are going to remain seated for this relaxation meditation which also introduces a *mudra*, or sacred hand gesture into the practice. We will explore the significance of *mudra* (which are sacred hand gestures) in chapter six, but for now, just adopt one of the following two mudras, depending on when you are practicing your yoga.

Morning practice: Chin Mudra

Rest the hands on your legs, just above your knees, with the palms facing up towards the ceiling. Bring the index finger of each hand in and curl it into the inside of the thumb to make a circle. Keep the other three fingers on each hand stretched out straight. This *mudra* works to open the chest area and so you may feel quite light and very receptive to your thoughts and feelings. It is known as the 'psychic gesture of consciousness' and we use it to welcome the energy and consciousness of the new day.

Evening practice: Jnana Mudra

Fold the index fingers into each thumb so that the tip of the fingers contacts the root base of the thumb. Stretch out the other three fingers on each hand and gently rest the hands, palms down, on the knees ready to start your meditation (shavanasana). This *mudra* is known as the 'psychic gesture of knowledge and works to calm and withdraw our subtle energy body ready for rest and sleep. Therefore, we use it at the end of the day.

Meditation

This introductory Kundalini yoga practice session has rebalanced and realigned the chakra energy centers and awakened the Kundalini energy that lies coiled and sleeping in the root or base chakra, Muladhara. Just as a daily shower cleanses your body in Kundalini yoga, we believe meditation works to cleanse your mind. It will rejuvenate you after a busy day, can help counter stress, and banish tiredness.

We will keep the mind focused during this mediation using the chant, *Sat Nam*, which we used earlier in this practice session. Chant, silent in your mind, *Sat* as you inhale and *Nam* as you exhale. Remember, in yoga, we only ever breathe through the nose, so keep your mouth closed.

Now close your eyes and bring your awareness to your breath. Breathe slowly into a count of four, hold the breath for four and slowly exhale to a count of four. Do this 10 times to help settle the breath into a slow and rhythmic pattern. Now you can focus on the chant instead of counting the breath.

As you meditate, tune in your body. What can you feel and where? Is there a stiffness in your neck? Do your knees ache. Does your throat feel scratchy? Simply notice how you feel in each part of your body and move on to the next observation.

You are going to sit, this first time, for 5-10 minutes in meditation, but the idea is to build this up over time so that you can comfortably manage a meditation of 30 minutes or more. Keep bringing your awareness back to the breath and use the *Sat Nam* chant to stay focused until the end of this part of your practice.

Peace Chant to end your first Kundalini yoga practice

Use this closing mantra to honor your truthful identity - your Higher Self - and to send blessings into the world, give thanks, roll away your mat, and start or end your day.

'Sat Nam. Namaste.'

As you roll away your yoga mat until it is time for your next practice session, really try to experience all the changes you can feel in both your physical body, your energy, and your feelings of spiritual connection.

Kundalini yoga, as we now know, is often called the yoga of awareness and you will have noticed the one repeated instruction throughout this practice was to take time after each posture or change to the pattern of breathing to notice its impact on your body, on your psyche, and your energy. Developing this awareness is every bit as important as perfecting the postures and knowing what the Sanskrit names mean!

Chapter Summary

- You have now had a taste of the power of a Kundalini practice and experienced the positive energy changes even simple postures can trigger.

- You have seen too how you can harness the breath to enhance the benefits of your Kundalini yoga practice.

- You may be a beginner, but you have now seen how individual this practice is; you decide how fast or slow, or how many repetitions you do.

In the next chapter, we will learn a little more about the significance of chanting and singing and *mudra* and *bandha* in a Kundalini yoga practice.

Chapter Five: Understanding the subtle energies we activate with Kundalini Breathwork

In yoga, we describe the subtle energy as *prana*, which can be taken to mean the life force. We cannot see or touch *prana* but as our practice and understanding deepen, we will feel and notice the physical, emotional, and spiritual changes that take place once we work with this energy.

The Kundalini energy itself is simply a powerful aspect of the pranic energy, *Prana Shakti*, that flows through the body, but unlike the rest of the pranic energy, Kundalini lies dormant at the base of the spine until something triggers its awakening. And as we have seen, Kundalini yoga starts that awakening process.

We use the breath to work with *prana* but *prana* and breath are not the same things. You can think of them as being aligned, which is why one can influence the other, but there are important differences. You can, for example, hold your breath and count to 10; you cannot ever hold your *prana* or stop it from moving about the body.

Pranayama is the yogic practice of working with the breath to connect to *prana* and, as you master its techniques, even direct *prana* to those parts of the body that need it most. This is a useful skill because *prana* - the mystical lifeforce - is both revitalizing and healing.

If you studied biology at school, then you may have a picture in your head of how you breathe. If you do it now - take a deep breath in - you will feel the lungs in your chest inflate to accommodate the influx of air and you may even feel the diaphragm muscle below your rib cage contract and flatten to allow for that expansion and to create a vacuum that draws air into the body. Now breathe out. Feel the diaphragm return to its normal dome shape, which allows the lungs to deflate and forces air out of the body. Put your hands on the sides of your body, just below your rib cage, and feel this happening in your own body.

So that is a crude description of the mechanics of human respiration — the airways, the lungs, the diaphragm, and all their workings to take oxygenated air in and send carbon dioxide out to keep you and your living tissues alive and thriving. So, one way you can try to understand the difference between breath and prana is that one (breath) is a life-sustaining system while the other is life-giving (*prana*). If you have ever been with someone as they die, you will have experienced the shut-down and departure of these two systems; first the breath and then something stranger which you cannot see but which you can now feel the absence of. It is more than the fact someone has stopped breathing. It is 'something else that has gone. It is *prana.*

The name itself is composed of two Sanskrit syllables *'pra'* meaning constant and *'na'* meaning movement. So, the word *'prana'* refers to something that is always on the move and according to Yoga science, this constant motion begins at the very moment of conception.

There are two types of this energy in the body; prana shakti, which refers to dynamic and vital energy, and prana chitti (or manas) shakti which refers to mental energy. This is important to understand because it means that for prana to reach every organ of the body there must be two distinct energy channels supplying them. And these are distinct subtle energy channels, so they are not the blood vessels used to bring oxygenated blood to these same organs.

Now let's learn a little about the subtle pranic energy network and by subtle, I mean invisible to both the naked eye and even to highly sophisticated medical scanning devices. This is because this energy system works through energy pathways or systems known as meridians, *nadis*, and chakras.

We have already explored the role and significance of the chakras in chapter one where we worked our way through the seven major chakras in the body to locate the dormant Kundalini Shakti energy in the root chakra, Muladhara, at the base of the spine. But what we did not talk about were the subtle (invisible) channels through which the pranic energy moved. You may already have heard of meridians too, since these are the same channels used by TCM (Traditional Chinese Medicine) practitioners in treatments such as acupuncture. The channels you are less likely to have come across unless you have practiced one of the other forms of yoga, are the nadis.

The Pranic Energy Network

The invisible pathways through which the pranic energy current flows around the body are known as *nadis*. These are not the same as nerves, which transmit signals around the body, or blood vessels which transport blood. Nerves relate to the physical body. Nadis relates to the pranic, vital body.

Instead of imagining a physical structure, you can imagine the *nadis* as more of a process and one that is in constant action. According to yogic texts, there are 72,000 nadis which all operate like a superhighway communications network to carry and send pranic energy back and forth to every part of the body. Happily, we do not need to know about all 72,000 channels but we need to know a little more about the three most important of these, which are:

- Ida nadi - the channel for mental energy

- Pingala nadi - the channel for vital (physical) energy

- Sushumna nadi - the channel for spiritual energy

All three nadis originate in the root chakra, Muladhara, which we now know is also home to Kundalini Shakti.

When we awaken the healing Kundalini energy and encourage it to rise through the chakra energy system, we are sending it up from the root chakra through pingala nadi. The pingala energy channel diverts first to the right side of the body and then moves over to the left-hand side, crossing the ida nadi at the juncture of each chakra. And ida does the opposite, flowing first from the root chakra to the left-hand side of the body and then crossing over to the right through each chakra.

These two subtle energy channels do this all the way up through the chakras and up through the body until they reach the 5th chakra, Anja chakra, or the Third Eye. Here, pingala, the vital energy stops.

Sushumna nadi, the channel for the spiritual energy, does not crisscross the body like the other two energy channels but rises straight up from the base chakra up through the center of each chakra. You can think of sushumna as the 'control' nadi. It is this channel that is the 'conductor' of Kundalini Shakti (energy) up through the body once it has awakened.

How to check your subtle body energy channels
Let's step away from the theory for a moment and do something that will not only tune you into your subtle energy channels but also reveal which one is dominant. In physical terms, the flow and function of the nadis are reflected in the flow of breath through your nostrils. You can now understand why, whenever we talk about a practice involving the breath, I take the trouble to remind you that in yoga; we breathe through the nose, not the mouth.

Take a moment now to close your eyes and observe the flow of your breath in and out of your nose. Notice that the flow is stronger in one nostril and be aware that one may even be partially blocked. This is because the ida and pingala nadis are only semi-active; sometimes one will work, sometimes the other. You can assess whether pingala is flowing from observing the breath flow in your right nostril and do the same with the left, which is related to ida activity.

If you spend a little time with this tuning-in exercise, you will notice the 'dominant' nostril changes, as does the breath flow. If the left nostril opens more, the flow in the right will reduce and even become blocked and vice versa.

Sometimes, both nostrils will be open and working optimally and when this is the case, this is a sign that sushumna is active.

Tuning into the Nadis

- Right nostril is dominant = pingala is active = you will feel more extroverted and energized

- Left nostril is dominant - ida is active = you will feel more tranquil, peaceful, and introverted

- Both nostrils are flowing and open = sushumna = you will feel calm, steady, and even more meditative

Nadi Shodhana- Alternate Nostril Breathing

This pranayama practice works on both the physical (gross) and subtle levels to improve general health and wellbeing and increase mental clarity. It delivers extra oxygen to all the tissues in the body and helps the lungs expel carbon dioxide more efficiently. It increases vitality and lowers stress and anxiety by harmonizing the pranic energy. In addition, the more you practice, the more it works to clear any prana blockages, to rebalance the pingala and ida energy channels, and support the flow of the subtle energies through sushumna nadi, leading to a deep a peaceful experience of your Kundalini practice, especially the mediation.

Hold the fingers of your right hand in front of your face.

Rest the index and middle fingers gently on the center of your forehead at the same level as your eyebrows. Keep all fingers relaxed.

Your thumb should now be at the same level as your right-hand nostril, and your little finger will be at the same level as your left-hand nostril. You are going to use your thumb and then the tip of your little finger to gently close and open each nostril to control the flow of your breath.

If you plan to practice for several minutes, you can support the elbow of your right arm with your left hand but take care not to block the front of the chest area.

Gently close the right nostril with the thumb and breathe in through the left nostril.

As you are breathing in count (in your head): "*1. Om. 2. Om. 3. Om*" until the inhalation ends.
Now close the left nostril with the tip of the little finger and allow the breath to flow out of the right nostril, counting (in your head): "*1. Om. 2. Om. 3. Om*" until the exhalation ends.

Repeat this by keeping the left nostril closed as you inhale through the right nostril counting (in your head): "*1. Om. 2. Om. 3. Om*" until the inhalation ends.

And then close the right nostril with the thumb, release the left and exhale through the left nostril counting (in your head): "*1. Om. 2. Om. 3. Om*" until the exhalation ends.

This counts as one round.

You can work on your alternate nostril breathing and build up to 10 rounds as part of your yoga practice.

The Psychic Breath & Ujjayi Breathing

This breathwork technique is the key to unlocking pranic healing and working with a Kundalini yoga practice to awaken Kundalini Shakti.

To understand the term, 'psychic breath' we simply mean you learn to integrate the physical breath with your awareness of prana and how it crisscrosses or moves up through the body through the nadis.

Ujjayi breathing and breathwork is the foundation of any serious yogic practice and if you join a class, you may already have seen someone else using this breathing technique to deepen their experience of the yoga practice.

The first step in mastering this technique is to do nothing at all, except to observe the natural rhythm of your 'gross' breathing right now. Gross, here, just means unsubtle. It is the physical respiration we can see and sometimes hear.

The fact is most of us breathe about 15 times a minute, paying no attention to the breath moving in and out of our bodies. It is something that just happens - 21,600 times over a 24-hour day.

A key part of any pranayama practice in yoga work is learning to first notice our breathing and then, second, to manipulate this 'gross' process through willpower, focus, and concentration.

Ujjayi breathing involves both the practice of awareness of the breath with a physical semi-contraction of the throat muscles. Once we master this (which will feel strange at first and take a little practice to get right) we realize the deep sound and vibration the breath makes as it both enters and leaves the body.

Ujjayi is a blissful practice because it works on both a physical (gross) level to calm and regulate the breath but also on a deeply spiritual level to connect us to a sense of tranquility, peace, and one-pointedness. We can then use ujjayi breathing to direct the 'psychic' breath and *prana*.

Ujjayi breathing is crucial in a Kundalini yoga practice because as we practice it, we begin, for the first time, to move the pranic energy at will. You will, likely, feel the first manifestation of this giant step forward as a tickling sensation in the throat, chest, and lungs. This sensation will pass. It simply shows that prana is moving in that region. If you are meditating, you may 'see' a stream of white light circling through the heart chakra in the center of your chest and firing off out to the body's organs and tissues surrounding it.

Do not rush any part of this practice or experience. Once you have discovered the power of ujjayi breathing, it will never leave you. You may abandon your yoga mat for years, but you will still slip into the psychic breath, especially when feeling increased stress like during a visit to the dentist or whatever feels stressful to you.

If you have a teacher, ask them to spend a little extra time with you to show ujjayi breathing and if not, have a look on YouTube because seeing someone else breathing this way can help remove any fear blocks that may stop you from mastering the technique.

The Psychic Passage
This concept is as important as all those we are exploring in this chapter because it will be a key part of your ability to successfully awaken and raise the Kundalini energy.

A psychic passage, in yoga, is any pathway through which you can direct the combination of awareness, breath, and *prana* as one combined stream/force. You can make these passages anywhere; from or to any part of the body and so this is how you can direct the healing pranic energy to those areas where it may be needed.

Once you have visualized the psychic passage, you can move the psychic breath anywhere in the body using your awareness and your ujjayi breathwork. This takes time, patience, and practice but if you commit to it, one day you will be on your yoga mat and realize this now happens spontaneously.

Chapter Summary

- We have learned more about the subtle energy pathways that crisscross the body and how there is a central pathway which will be the route the Kundalini energy takes when it rises.

- We have learned two new pranayama techniques that are crucial for learning to control the movement of prana around the body.

- We have discovered the importance of ujjayi breathing, which also works to connect us to a more deeply spiritual yoga practice.

In the final chapter, we will learn a little more about the significance of both *bandha* and *mudra* in a Kundalini yoga practice.

Chapter Six: Kundalini You

The subtle thread of the spirit can expand and contract within the body. When it expands, it passes through the brain, heart, and body to experience life, and when the same subtle thread of the spirit is taken inwardly, it contracts itself into the soul, to experience the bliss from within."
-Roshan Sharma

If there's one thing we can state categorically, it is that a Kundalini yoga practice can be a life experience that may come as a surprise, especially to those used to a more sedate practice.

The powerful breathwork, for example, we have just described in the previous chapter plus the use of mantra, chanting, singing, and sometimes even running and jumping will awaken 'something' in you. You will feel more creative, more inspired, more confident, and more productive. Remember how at the start of the book, we talked about Kundalini yoga's aim of helping you to connect to a different version of you: your Higher Self if you like. Well, I forgot to mention how much 'bigger' this new person is.

But alongside the breathwork, the chanting, and the singing, two of the yogic techniques that Kundalini yoga places great emphasis on are mudra and bandha. You've now had a very basic introduction to both through the suggested daily practice outlined in chapter four, so here, we will dive a little more into their spiritual significance.

Yogic Energy Locks - Bandha

The Sanskrit word, *Bandha*, means to hold, to tighten, or to lock. So, in very simple terms, the practice of bandha is used to hold or lock the pranic energy in a particular part of the body and redirect its flow into sushumna nadi for spiritual awakening. We understand now that Kundalini Yoga is said to be the most spiritual form of all the yoga practices (all that means is there is a more overt spiritual emphasis that may lack in other classes), so *bandha* is important to us.

You can practice *bandhas* individually or incorporate them into mudra and pranayama practices where they can help awaken the psychic faculties and build a stronger bridge to the 'higher' more spiritual yogic practices.

There are four distinct bandhas; *jalandhara, moola* (which we practiced in chapter four) *uddiyana*, and *maha*, the last being a combination of the first three locks.

The *bandhas* act upon something called *granthis*, which are referred to as psychic knots. Here you can see which bandha works on which psychic knot:

- Moola Bandha acts on Brahma Granthi

- Uddiyana Bandha acts on Vishnu Granthi

- Jalanhandra Bandha acts on Rudra Granthi

It is the granthis (psychic knots) that prevent the free flow of prana along the sushumna nadi and thus impede the awakening chakras and the rising of Kundalini Shakti. What this tells us then, is that learning and practicing the bandha energy locks is a critical part of a successful Kundalini practice, otherwise the Kundalini energy may awaken but cannot ascend.

The Granthis and what they govern

Brahma granthi: This is the 1st psychic knot and is linked with the root and sacral chakras, Muladhara and Swadhisthana (revisit chapter one to refresh your memory about the location and function of these energy centers). This is the region concerned with the survival instinct, the urge to procreate, our instincts, and deeper desires. Once this psychic knot is transcended, kundalini can rise beyond these desires, without the risk of it being pulled back down by the attractions and preferences of the earthbound personality.

Vishnu granthi: This is the 2nd psychic knot and is linked with the manipura and anahata, the sacral and the heart chakras. These two chakras are concerned with the sustenance of the physical, emotional, and mental aspects of our existence and so govern processes such as digestion. Once this knot is transcended, Kundalini can rise and beyond these chakras and the yogi can now draw collective consciousness and energy from the universe, rather than localized centers within the human body itself.

Rudra granthi: This is the 3rd and final psychic knot and is associated with anja (also known as the Third Eye) and the crown (vishuddi) chakras which are concerned with the higher spiritual levels of thinking. When Kundalini can transcend this psychic knot, the ego is shattered and dropped, and we become one with the whole. This also explains why a Kundalini practice is sometimes known as '**The Ego Slayer.**'

Jalandhara Bandha

This is also known as the throat lock. It can help relieve stress and anxiety and on a physical level, can keep the sinus passages clear and healthy.

1. Sit cross-legged on your mat and use a yoga roll or cushion to raise your hips so that your knees keep contact with the floor if that is more comfortable for you.

2. Put your palms on your knees.

3. Close your eyes and try to relax the entire body.

4. Inhale, slowly and deeply, and hold the breath inside.

5. Tip the head forward and press your chin into the top of your chest.

6. Straighten the arms and keep them straight by pressing your palms firmly onto your knees.

7. Hunch the shoulders up and forward which works to apply more pressure to the neck region.

8. Stay in this; position for as long as you can hold your breath. but don't strain the body.

9. Relax the shoulders and gently release the bandha throat lock as you raise the head, exhale, and release the breath you have been holding inside.

10. Allow your breathing to return to normal and then repeat twice more.

11. You can build up slowly to a round of 10 repetitions.

Contraindications: Do not practice this bandha if you have high blood pressure or heart disease.

Uddiyana Bandha*

We have already tried moola bandha so let's try uddiyana bandha which, as we have just learned, works on the second of the psychic knots and allows Kundalini to rise to help sustain us in our more spiritual and less earthly concerns. You can also think of this bandha as being a powerful abdominal contraction.

Sit on your yoga mat in a comfortable cross-legged position. (Raise your hips by sitting on a yoga roll or cushions to allow the knees to rest on the mat which might be more comfortable if you are not used to crossed-legged sitting for any period.)

1. Place the palms of the hands flat on the knees and draw the spine up so it is straight.

2. Close the eyes and relax the entire body.

3. Breath in deeply through the nostrils and exhale through the mouth with a whoosh' to try to empty the lungs as much as you can

4. Hold the breath outside the body

5. Lean forward, press down on the knees with the palms of the hands. Straighten the elbows and raise the shoulders which will help extend the spine into a stretch.

6. Drop your chin down to press into your chest

7. Now, contract the abdominal muscles inwards and upwards.

8. Hold this abdominal lock (bandha) and keep the breath outside the body for as long as you can but don't strain the body.

9. Now, release the abdominal muscles, bend the elbows and lower the shoulders back to a normal resting position.

10. Raise the head, slowly inhale and allow the breath to return to normal before repeating the *bandha.*

11. Repeat twice more and, over time, build up to a round of 10 repetitions.

Beginner's Tip: *This bandha is easier to practice if preceded by an inverted asana. It can be a powerful experience so do not rush it. Be sure to stop if you feel nauseous or upset. You should also only try this bandha on an empty stomach and having emptied your bowels.*

Contraindications: Do not practice this bandha if you have high blood pressure or heart disease or if you are pregnant.

Maha bandha, which is a combination of the three locks you have now experienced, is an advanced practice and is not recommended for beginners.

The Joy of Mudras

I have already introduced you to two different *mudras* (sacred hand gestures) in our practice session in chapter four where I promised we would delve a little more deeply, at the end of the book (here) into why they are important and how they can enhance our Kundalini Yoga practice once we incorporate them.

The Sanskrit word mudra means hand gesture, and in Kundalini Yoga, mudras are often used as a sign of devotion to the yogic tradition, plus a way of linking our pranic energy to the universal or cosmic force.

The etymological root of the word *mudra* is *mud* which translates to 'delight' or 'pleasure' and the second syllable, *dravay* or *dru* which means 'to draw forth.' So, this tells us we can use *mudra* in our Kundalini Yoga practice to 'draw forth' delight or if you prefer, joy!

Mudras are usually subtle, physical gestures or movements which we can use in yoga to alter mood, perception, and even our attitude, all of which can help to deepen our awareness and connection to the spiritual aspects of our practice and our emerging Higher Self.

A mudra can involve the entire body in a combination of asana, pranayama, bandha, and meditation, or they can be a simple hand gesture that nobody who was not aware of their significance would even notice.

Traditionally, mudras were never described in written texts but were handed from guru to student when the latter was deemed proficient enough and ready to receive the wisdom of *mudra*. And what is agreed among practitioners is that they are higher practices that are used to lead to the awakening of the *prana* energy (life force), the chakras, and the Kundalini serpent energy - all of which can give significant psychic powers to the advanced yogi.

The study of *mudra* is, therefore, also an advanced study but even for a beginner and someone new to Kundalini Yoga, it's helpful to understand a little more because, even in a beginner's class, your teacher will probably introduce you to both hands and head mudras. We have already tried, both here and in our practice session in chapter four, the *bandha mudras* so you are already no stranger to the importance and practice of *mudra*.

What may still surprise you is that the part of the body that even the simplest of mudras works on is the brain and not just the brain, but those primitive parts around the brain stem which govern our unconscious reflexes and primal, instinctual habits and patterns.

In some mysterious way, *mudras* simply bypass the intellect to establish a subtle connection with this ancient part of your brain to create a link which then can have a corresponding impact on your body, your mind, and the prana that we know is always in a constant state of flux and movement.

And so, the aim when we practice *mudra,* is for these fixed and repetitive postures and gestures to snap us out of old patterns and behaviors. By doing so, they help us establish a more yogic and refined consciousness that is more in keeping with our Higher Self and its spiritual and worldly preferences.

In chapter four, I introduced you to both *chin mudra* and *jnana mudra* as part of your meditation and mudra practice. What I can share now is that those mudras which join the thumb and the index fingers in this way engage the brain and our sensory/motor functions subtly by generating a loop of energy that flows from the brain down to the hand and back up again.

I don't have the science to prove this to you, but that doesn't much matter because I don't need it. If you practice *mudra* and start with these simple but powerful sacred hand gestures, you will experience what I am describing here for yourself. Try it next time you step onto your yoga mat and see for yourself what I am describing and just how powerful it is. The other thing we know from our awareness of our practice is the more you use *mudra,* the more powerful it becomes.

Mana - Head Mudras
Your Kundalini practice will include mana, or head mudras, which are integral to this highly spiritual yoga discipline. These are so effective and so powerful that many form a simple meditation in their own right. They can use the eye, the ears, the nose, the tongue, or the lips. Here is simple technique that uses the nose - *nasi* means nose - and is perfect for beginners to try:

Nasikagra Drishti (nose tip gazing)

1. Sit on your yoga mat in any comfortable meditation position that allows you to keep the spine straight.
2. Rest the hand on the knees in *chin* (palms facing up, daytime) or *jnana* (palms facing down, night time) *mudra.*

3. Close your eyes and relax your body.

4. Now, open your eyes and focus them on the very tip of your nose.

5. Do not strain the eyes but try to keep them relaxed.

6. When you achieve the correct focus a double outline of the nose appears and these two lines converge at the tip of the nose to create an inverted 'V' shape.

7. Focus on the point of this upside-down 'V.'

At first, this practice will feel difficult. You may feel a headache threatening, so start slowly.

Eventually, you can slowly build up to gazing at the tip of your nose for five or even 10 minutes at a time. And although your eyes are open throughout, this is an introspective practice that takes your attention away from the outside world and external events and brings it inside, thus creating introspection. The whole idea is for you to use this simple but initially demanding *mudra* practice to help you transcend normal awareness.

Focusing on the tip of the nose concentrates the mind and the more you practice, the more you will experience the multiple benefits of *Nasikagra Drishti* which include dispelling anger and calming the mind. We also use this *mudra* in Kundalini Yoga because it helps to awaken the root chakra - Muladhara - at the base of the spine which is where Kundalini Shakti also lives!

If you are wondering how this works when the tip of the nose is, physically, nowhere near the base of the spine where you will find Muladhara chakra, then the explanation lies because symbolically, with *nashikagra drishti,* the bridge of the nose is related to the spinal cord. At the top, you have the eyebrow center - Ajna chakra or the Third Eye - and at the bottom, which in this analogy is the tip of the nose, Muladhara or the root chakra which is then activated because by gazing at the tip of the nose you are also gazing into this chakra center.

Khechari Mudra (Tongue lock)

This is another deceptively simple mudra that will also leave you feeling calm once you have mastered it.

1. Sit on your yoga mat in any comfortable meditation position that allows you to keep the spine straight.

2. Rest the hand on the knees in *chin* (palms facing up, daytime) or *jnana* (palms facing down, night time) *mudra.*

3. Close your eyes and relax your body.

4. Now, fold your tongue upward and backward so that the lower surface contacts the roof of your mouth.

5. Do not strain to achieve this but allow it to happen.

6. If you have mastered it, you are now going to start *ujjayi pranayama* (see chapter five for detailed instructions on how to do this)

7. Breathe slowly and deeply and hold the breath inside for as long as you can before slowly exhaling.

8. Your tongue will soon feel tired so when this happens, relax it, take a brief break, and repeat the mudra.

This *mudra* is all about inner healing. When the tongue contacts the top of the mouth, it stimulates the secretion of hormones and saliva on the physical level. But on the metaphysical, when it is combined with *ujjayi pranayama* it helps us to develop greater awareness of the psychic passages (see chapter five) that relate to the spine.

So, ultimately, this powerful *mudra* has the potential to stimulate prana and awaken Kundalini Shakti.

Chapter Summary

- We have learned there are three energy locks or bandhas that we use in our Kundalini yoga practice to remove the 'blocks' that would otherwise prevent the Kundalini energy from rising.

- We have been introduced to the highly spiritual significance of *mudra* in bypassing our intellect to communicate with our brain and our Higher Self.

- We have learned how important both head and hand mudras are in a Kundalini Yoga practice because they can be used, with care and awareness, to help awaken the Kundalini energy.

Conclusion

I hope you've enjoyed learning about Kundalini, and feel ready to begin your own Kundalini Yoga practice. Whether you decide to go this path alone, or wish to enroll in a Kundalini class, you should now feel as though you have a good understanding of what the practice is about, how it works, and what you stand to achieve from it.

Thank you for taking the time to read this book. I wish you the best of luck in your spiritual journey!

*"May the long-time sun
Shine upon you,
All love surround you,
And the pure light within you
Guide your way on."*

- Kundalini Yoga farewell blessing

www.ingramcontent.com/pod-product-compliance
Lightning Source LLC
LaVergne TN
LVHW021738060526
838200LV00052B/3346